Tips and Techniques to Heal and Prevent Backaches Naturally

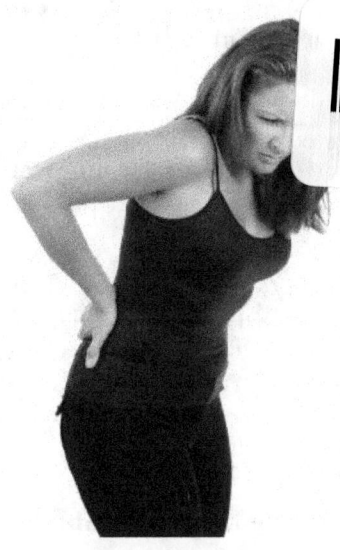

Dueep Jyot Singh

Healthy Learning Series

Mendon Cottage Books

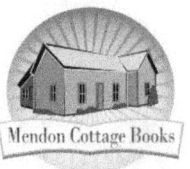

JD-Biz Publishing

Download Free Books!

http://MendonCottageBooks.com

Our books are available at

1. Amazon.com
2. Barnes and Noble
3. Itunes
4. Kobo
5. Smashwords
6. Google Play Books

Download Free Books!

http://MendonCottageBooks.com

Table of Contents

Introduction

Did you know that one of the most common of human ailments is the one to which anybody can fall prey anywhere – a backache! A tired child is going to complain of backache, if it has spent the whole day over exerting the muscles of the back. You are going to suffer from backache, if you happened to pick up a heavy box the wrong way, and then got up with a jerk and found that twinge affecting your back. And as you grow older and older, you may suffer age-related backache problems.

This book is going to tell you all about tips and techniques with which you can prevent backaches, heal backaches, and also how a little bit of common sense can help you make sure that your whole life is backache free.

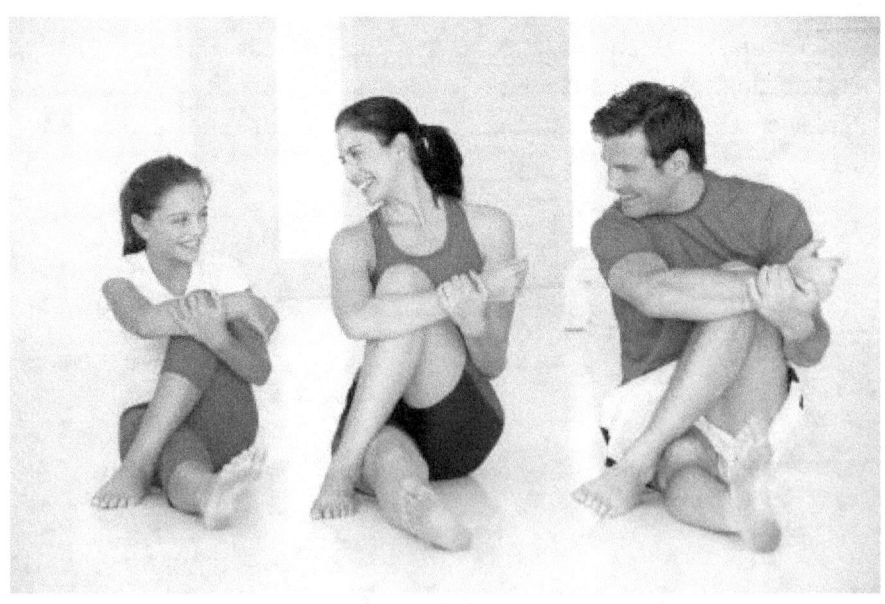

Healthy back muscles from childhood onwards mean no backaches ever.

Naturally, having led a childhood and youthful of lots of physical exercises, especially during physical training sessions at school and university, there was absolutely no chance of us suffering from backache ever.

And if anybody asked is the reason for such a phenomena, naturally we would think for a second and decide that that was because all our muscles were properly exercised, and limber. The root cause for all the back pain and literal pain in the neck is weak muscles of the spine.

During our early morning 7 o'clock physical training sessions during our cadet Corps training at University, any sort of physical activity and PT always began with back stretches. Our trainer, Major A. soon found out that we high spirited over- exuberant and thoroughly lighthearted potential juvenile delinquents enjoyed these sessions very much, because the stretching exercises for us were more like parodies of Bollywood dance moves in choreographic order!

So when she asked us to stretch our hands above our heads, and do backward stretches, all of us put on dance poses, doing our version of happy dances, with rhythmic hips swaying movements, and a bit of ad-libbed dancing.

She was a good sport, even though she told us often, mouth grim, but eyes twinkling, that she was not training us to be future movie stars, but future star athletes and healthy young things! Nevertheless, back pain was a quantity unknown to us. And to think of it, we never suffered from morning body aches, stiffness, back pain when we bent and other problems of the back.

You may say that we were just teenagers and at that particular age, backaches are rare. But I think it was because of our simple and healthy lifestyles, with lots of games, exercise [*or our version of dancing*], especially in the open air.

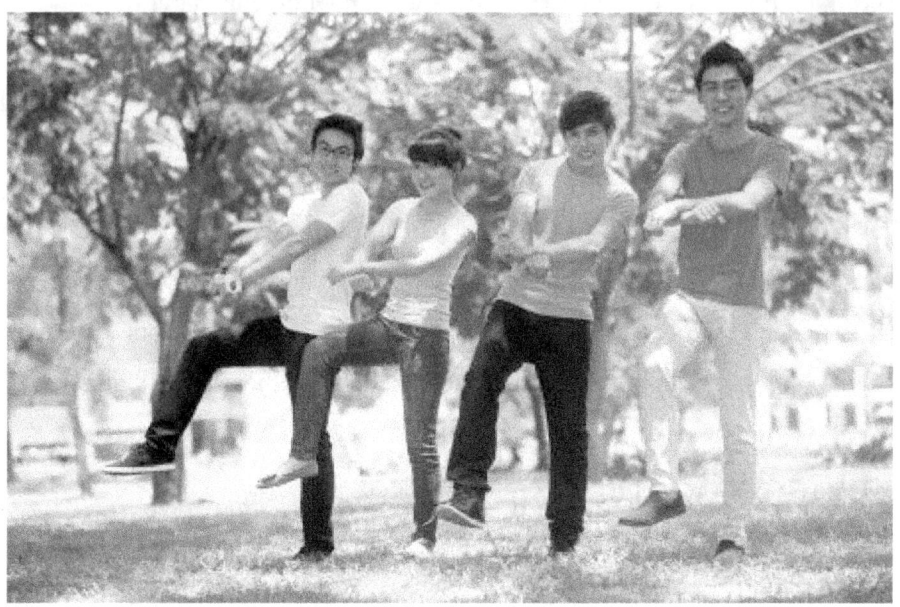

Just imagine, thinking of exercising for 15 minutes is enough to make you break into a figurative and literal sweat, but the idea of dancing for half an hour at a stretch does not make you shudder at all, because that comes under the jolly good fun part of life! This is all in the mind and psyche and an integral part of human psychology.

It is only later I understood why she never lost her temper with us, even though the supposed exercises that we were doing were definitely not in any military training manual!

The ad lib dance routines into which we went, for hours on end, were strenuous enough to exercise each and every muscle in our bodies, while traditional and conventional set routines of PT exercises just said *Hup - 1 – 2 – 3 – 4, 5 – 6 – 7 – 8 – repeat that session again, 1... And so on. A*nd these definitely did not go in for any sort of spontaneous exercising/training of other sets of muscles!

Later on when we grew up and began piloting desks, most of us suffered from backaches, because of a large number of reasons. Along with this, most of us suffered from neck pain, and spinal problems. One of the main reasons was bad posture.

Bad Posture

I do not know how and where you are sitting, reading this book on your Kindle. If you are slumped on your bed, just look at the way you have managed to tuck in your shoulders and slouched, with your stomach all accordioned in and almost touching your chest.

The Victorians were very particular about posture, and that is why they always made sure that the back was always straight, especially when they stood or sat down. Unfortunately, that stiff back attitude made sure that they suffered from stiff necks, because the neck was not given enough of exercise or leeway in order to move about. But they considered that poster to be ladylike or even gentleman – like. And thus, the term, stiffnecked, pompous, priggish, and a bore.

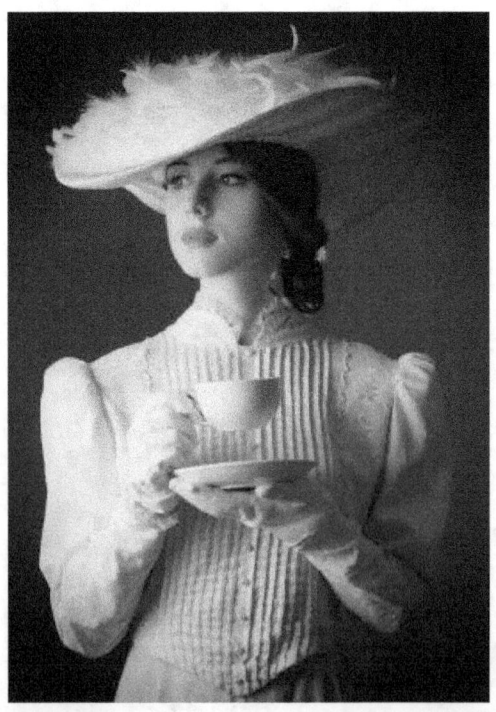

I remember as a student at college, being beaten regularly – not a painful caning, but an admonishing whip just to remind me, across my shoulders by the good Major – we thoroughly admired her and liked her very much. So we accepted her strict discipline – who kept telling me not to slouch like a vulture and straighten my shoulders proudly. She did not want me to become a future hunchback!

So, the moment I began to slouch, zip went her rattan cane across the shoulders, and stand up straight! I immediately used to stiffen up, and then she used to yell, do not stiffen up your neck, also at the same time, let it fall loose. And naturally, tuck your stomach and behind in, and put your chin up.

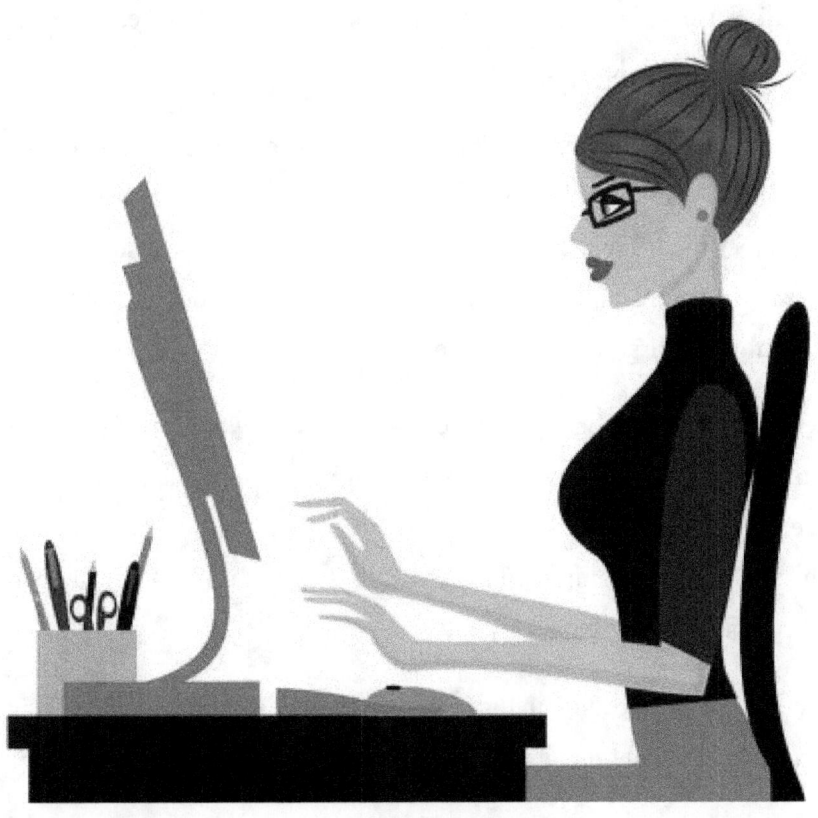

I did that until the moment she was out of sight, and then went loose muscled again – a slouch is always so much easier! Nevertheless, three years of this training had me walking properly, with all the muscles coordinated, and later on, when I was training professional models, they had to learn to walk correctly before they learned anything else.

I had to get rid of my stalking tiger like lope, 1 foot purposely placed before the other and marching right ahead, in order to teach them the best way to walk!

The easiest way and of course the correct way was to swing from the hips and definitely not from the knees. The toes were pointed in the same direction and they had to learn never to walk with their toes pointing outwards. Have you seen the Native Americans and also Africans walk? They walk correctly – ever so slightly pigeon toed. It is very healthy for your feet, and it also looks better.

For this, my professional model /trainer friend, from whom I learned the correct way of walking told me – just draw a line on the floor. Now, place 1 foot with toes facing forward on the line. Swing the other foot/leg with exaggerated gestures, in initial stages from the hip, with the heel of the other foot touching the first toe of the 1st foot.

Incidentally, when she had her classes, all of us who were free, faculty, and also students use to come and look at these practice sessions, because we were learning to walk like professional models. Later on, we faculty members would be teaching them, especially those of us who already had some previous modeling background.

And soon, it began to come natural, and we did not even have to use a chalk line. We just looked at the ground, saw that it was straight, and level, and then began walking, slightly fast, rather than slow, walking slightly fast keeps the rhythm level. And thanks to this walk, it looked like we knew where we were going, and we went there proudly!

Obesity and Back Problems

You may not know this, but if you are suffering from a weight problem, there is a chance that you are going to suffer from back problems. Also, if you are underweight, there is a chance that your spinal cord is going to become weaker, because of bad muscular coordination, and weak tissues.

So how is this way of pigeon toed walking going to help your back problem? All the weight of the body is going to be distributed equally, when your feet are placed correctly on the ground. You are going to suffer from back problems, if you have an obesity problem.

That means there is too much weight put on your feet. That means they are getting tired. That means that you are going to be leaning forward in order to get some of the weight off your feet. So you cannot walk lightly, but you are going to be clomping all over the place, even though some obese people are really light on their feet, especially when they are dancing.

So what is the correct posture, you are going to say? Your back should never be stiff, nor should your neck. Just stand up straight, and let all the muscles and your spinal cord fall naturally into place. That is the natural position of where the muscles are supposed to be, and make sure that you do not stand in any pose/posture, where these muscles do not fall naturally.

Proper Back Support

Neckache?

Once upon a time, I suffered terribly from backaches and even from potential spondylitis, because I used to sit crouched up before a computer for hours, without moving. Many of us, with such particular lifestyles are going to suffer from stiff muscles, and an aching back, when they get up from a session in front of a computer.

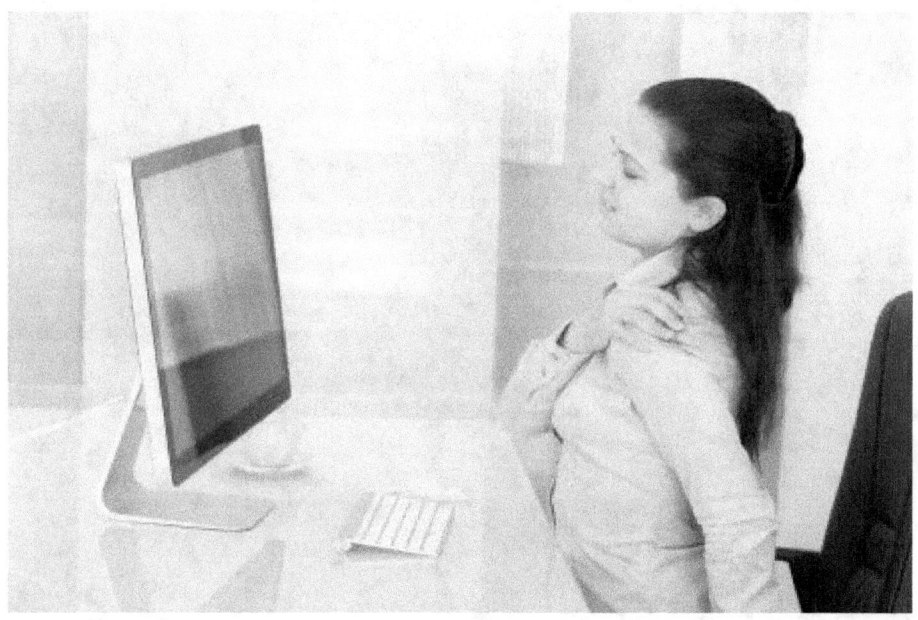

Doctors say that using chairs that have a fixed back support and an inclination between 90 – 110° are good for your back. You need to sit on a chair which has the proper back support with your hips all the way behind and your legs supported flat right on the floor. This is going to ensure that the pressure of your body is distributed equally throughout your spine.

Well, I tried it out. That did not work too good for me, especially as I wanted a chair on which I could lean back, when thinking on what to write next and how to word it.

So this is what I decided, in order to keep my spine straight, neck moving easily, and also lots of support to the small of my back. This is a picture of my computer chair. It is an ordinary garden chair with arms supports on which I can rest my arms and hands.

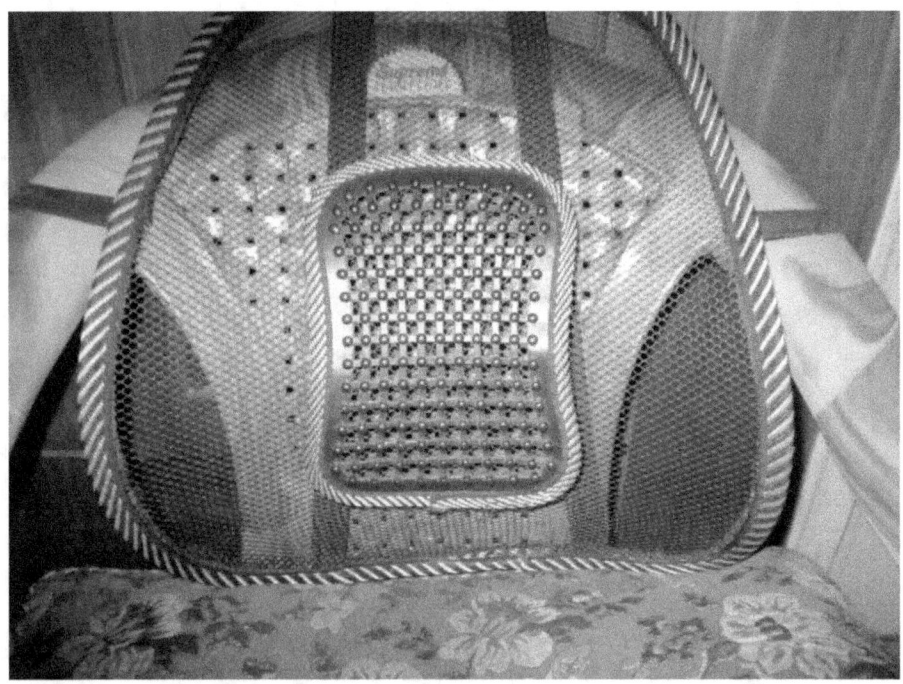

The soft cushion is just because I like to sit on soft cushions, even if I "am not eating strawberries and cream and sewing a fine seam."

Attached to the back of the chair is a backrest from our car. These are getting to be the in thing in our country, being sold at every crossroads by street urchins, at the nominal price of equivalent to one dollar. I do not know which particular car company decided that this was a good idea – attachments – for drivers going on long-term drives, but I decided that if it could support their backs, it could support mine, especially when I was also sitting for hours on end!

Seriously speaking, this experiment has worked so well that I have suggested this idea to all my friends and relatives, especially when they have the habit of sitting in front of a computer.

And when I switch off the computer, and it is time to relax and recuperate at night, semi – lying in bed and just reading or listening to music/audiobooks, I just remove this back support and put it around my back – supporting pillow! No chance of backaches ever.

You may want to try it out right now. Contact your nearest car dealer!

You are going to ask why this works wonders for your back. That is because the design of this support pays a lot of attention to the curvature of the spine. One of the key points in keeping the spine limber, especially with a lumbar support helps prevent backache and muscular stiffness and pain.

If you find yourself sitting on beanbags or on sofas that are too soft, you are going to suffer from potential back problems because the spinal cord does not get adequate support. Also sitting on a chair cross-legged for a number of hours results in stiff muscles and a backache, because your posture is too stiff and your muscles are not being allowed much leeway and movement.

Sitting on the floor, especially in tight jeans and trousers, was a normal pastime for a number of us, especially at college, but without any back support, and for a long time, we would possibly suffer from a backache. Especially when we got up to stretch our legs after a number of hours – ooh,aah - ouch- and found our backs stiff.

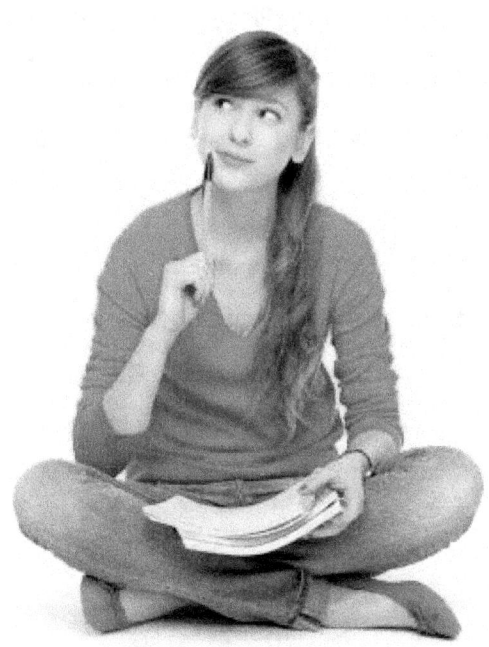

However, nowadays, we are so used, to not exercising or doing anything to strengthen our spinal cord and back muscles that slowly and steadily, the muscles give away. This is going to lead to a lot of stress on the spine in the future.

So if you are trying some strengthening exercises, especially under the close supervision of a professional, make sure that any sort of work out is begun with warm-up exercises and ended with cooling down exercises.

If you have a weak mid region, especially an underdeveloped core, do not try any high-end activities like lifting heavy weights.

How to Prevent Spine Stress

We use all our muscles for all the goodies during our daily work sessions, but we do not do anything to strengthen them. That is why, when you are sitting at work, it is good to do a few stretching exercises when you are sitting at your desk. Take frequent breaks from constant desktop work, get up, and move about around the room to work your spinal muscles which may have stiffened in the interim.

Doing the Cat Stretch

I learned this trick from watching cats, especially the exercise they did the moment they got up. Firstly, they stretched their limbs to the utmost, front and back limbs. Then they loosened their back muscles to get rid of all the muscular and tissue kinks, which had been brought about during their sleep and rest.

The cat stretch is done very, very slowly, without any jerky movements. You are going to stretch every part of your back slowly and steadily, until you find the muscles loosening. If you find yourself waking up with back pain, the moment you get up, it means that you have been sleeping in one particular position, throughout the night – flat on your back. Be like a cat, curl up, with your spinal cord curved.

And when you get up, you are going to stretch every muscle in your body in every direction. Just think that you are reaching out for something just beyond your reach. The movement should not be jerky. If you feel any sort of pain anywhere, be very careful, because it may possibly be your body's way of signaling to you that there is something wrong somewhere. And this signal is most important, especially if you get it first thing in the morning, the moment you wake up, and especially when it is recurrent. In such a case, you are not going to ignore it, and you will have to look at the underlying cause of such discomfort.

Let me give you my example. A month or two ago, I used to wake up from a not so healthy sleep, gasping for breath, and with a rip roaring headache. Thanks to this, I found my temper, as well as my health being affected. And the solution was so simple that many of us did not think about it. It was winter time and I had closed all the windows of the room. There was not enough oxygen, and no wonder I was suffering from headaches, due to a carbon dioxide buildup, during my rest.

So the very next night, even though the temperature was below -5°C, I left a window open, piled on the quilts, switched on the electric blanket, covered myself up thoroughly and cocooned myself against draughts and slept like a baby.

So the solution to all your problems are right there, if you use a little bit of logic and common sense.

Sleep – Healthy Restorer of Health

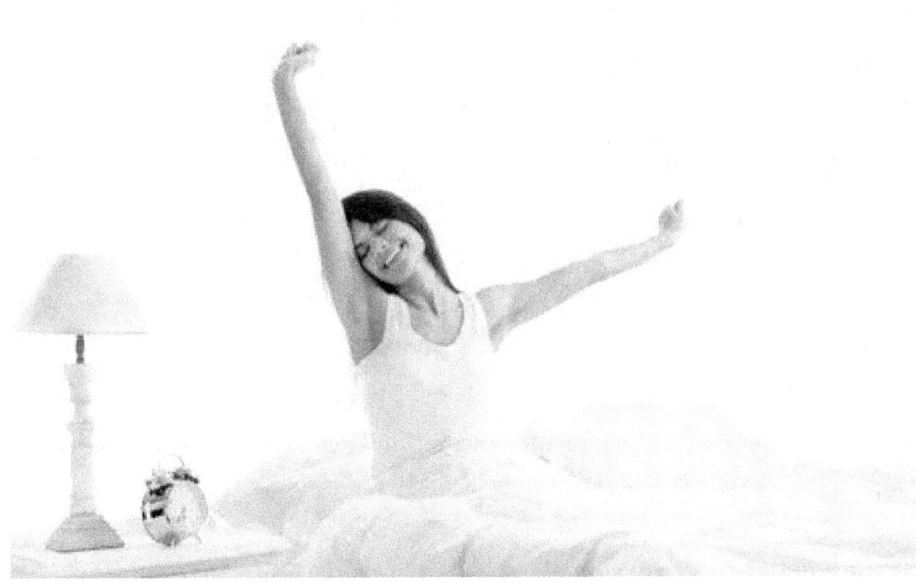

I was just laughing and telling a friend of mine who is a psychologist, that she has got people so afraid with Freudian psychoanalytic babble, that they have forgotten how to sleep, naturally. According to her, anybody who is curled up on his side – which is actually the natural way of sleeping, and our ancestors followed it – is psychologically afraid, insecure, and other such negative psychological, emotional problems.

When I told her that her suggestion that a healthy person is going to sleep flat on his back, with minimum movement, and that shows a healthy body and mind and psyche, he was just adding to potential back problems. That was because he was forcing his subconscious mind to straighten out, because the Doctor said so. So are you sleeping or forcing yourself to sleep with your back completely straight, limbs completely straight, and absolutely no curve anywhere in your body, and also not sleeping on your side, because the Doctor said that that was not a healthy sign, emotionally, or psychologically, forget what the doctor said.

This doctor is also going to tell you not to use pillows. I would rather you use pillows, that support the natural curve of your neck. Such a pillow should be just firm enough to induce sleep. When you are looking for mattresses, look for the one which suits you best, cotton or foam mattresses.

He is just making sure that you come to him with lots of back pain in the future. That is because he has taught you *how not to sleep properly!*

If your natural instinct says curl up, when you are half asleep, do that immediately and turn on your side. – and forget all the subconscious Freudian connotations, suggestions and implications – a little knowledge is a dangerous thing – curl up, especially if you are holding onto a pillow between your legs and clutching it as a security blanket.

Our ancestors did it on the treetops, and they were absolutely not pestered with any idiotic idea that this was not the proper way to sleep. If they had stretched out on the branches and gone off to sleep on their backs, they would have rolled off their perches or fallen prey to any predator hunting in the night! Later on, when human beings became more civilized and began to sleep on beds, they use to sleep on hard beds due to the necessity to sleep lightly.

A Proper Mattress

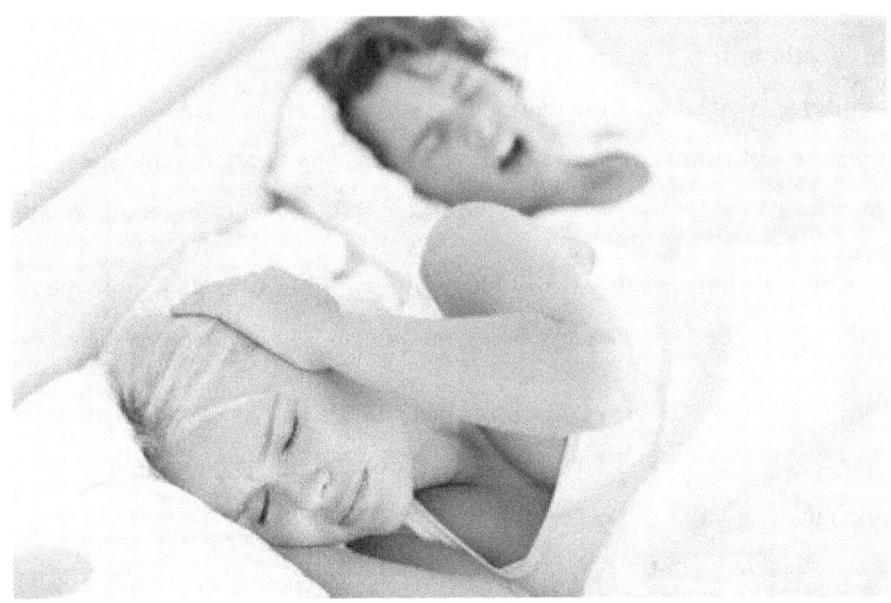

Apart from snoring, too hard a mattress or too soft a mattress can also be the cause of chronic insomnia, and too many sleepless nights. Incidentally, he is snoring, because he is lying on his back and his air passage is being obstructed. If he were sleeping on his side, he would not be snoring.

But nowadays, we have soft mattresses and hard mattresses. I have a number of friends who sleep on hard boards, because they have been brought up that way. And all of them suffer from backaches. That is because there is no leeway for the spinal cord to curve naturally on a hardboard. The same thing goes for a really hard mattress because that is equivalent to sleeping on an iron bench! And if the mattress is too soft, you were plenty of leeway for spinal curvature, but not enough back support.

So make sure that the coverings of your bed in the shape of mattresses are exactly right to support your spinal cord, give it plenty of proper curvature and also soft enough to promote a good night's sleep.

In ancient times, it was only the Saints and Wise men, who used to sleep on the ground, because they considered this to be a way of life. The bed that one uses has to be firm. Sleeping on a very hard surface like on the floor or an extra hard mattress, however much the doctor suggests it is going to be detrimental to the health of your spine.

If the bed is not comfortable, you are going to wake up with a backache.

Incidentally, let me give you an example here. My father found himself suffering from back problems, about 30 years ago and the doctor asked him about the bed on which he was sleeping. This was an informal discussion, because my father had not been to a hospital since 1959, when he met with an accident.

My father said that it was a soft, traditional bed made of a frame, on which were woven tape rolls, covered with a couple of mattresses, and then bed linen.

So the doctor asked him if the woven tape roll had been retightened within the past couple of years on the bed frames!

It had not been, and it was all loose, not giving adequate support to the body. In fact, one could almost say that it was as loose as a hammock. So my grandmother taught us youngsters how the tape roll needed to be tightened on the wooden frame by pulling the warp and the weave of the tape roll, – my brother pulling the tape on top of the frame and I pulling its corresponding tape at the bottom of the frame – tightening it and safety pinning the left over roll, to one end of the weave, underneath at the end of the tightening session.

After that frame was replaced on the bed, back went on his traditional cotton mattresses and his linen, and father was never bothered about backaches again.

Until a decade later, when another doctor who was trying out his own theories, told him that he was doing harm to himself by sleeping on a woven bed roll and he had better sleep on a hard wooden plank.

Father took his advice for just three days, and it is a possibility that the mattresses were not soft enough. The fourth day he got up in agony, with a really stiff back, which had to be massaged back into place, with warm oil and plenty of pounding and pummeling.

That hard wooden plank was immediately turned into a table, waste not want not!

In ancient times, and even medieval times, the people who could afford them slept on goose feather beds. However, their beds were made of planks of wood. So the goose feathers were to give support to the body, while the planks of the wood were there to make sure that the sleeper did not go crashing down, to the ground, at night.

In ancient Europe, especially in cold regions like the Scandinavian countries, the whole family slept on heated platforms, which were made of clay or brick. They were then covered with fur and cloth, underneath and over them. And the next morning they got up and did a good day's work outside, exercising every stiff muscles, so there was no question of any sort of backache.

Also, they were very particular about their diet, eating a very rich high-protein diet and drinking plenty of liquids. Most of us have forgotten how to drink healthy liquids and we do not know that our intervertebral discs contain a large percentage of water. So if you are dehydrated, water loss is going to make those discs weaker. So plenty of water all the time and liquids for nourishment is imperative to have a healthy spinal cord.

In ancient times, diets included items with plenty of vitamin D3, vitamin B-12, and calcium in order to keep the spine and all the bones healthy. Most of the foods that we today does not have these vitamins because either they have been processed away, or we are encouraged to eat artificial supplements.

So for plenty of calcium, you need to eat eggs, drink plenty of milk, green vegetables for vitamin B12 and for vitamin D3, you are going to get them in fatty fish, omega-3 rich fish oils, cheese, egg yolk, liver, especially that of beef and fresh mushrooms. Also, this vitamin is available in sunshine, so remember to go out in the sun – at least once a day – in order to have healthy bones, healthy teeth, and healthy tissue muscles! Cholecalciferol, vitamin D3 is found in halibut, mackerel, salmon, trout, and even in lard and spareribs!

Massage

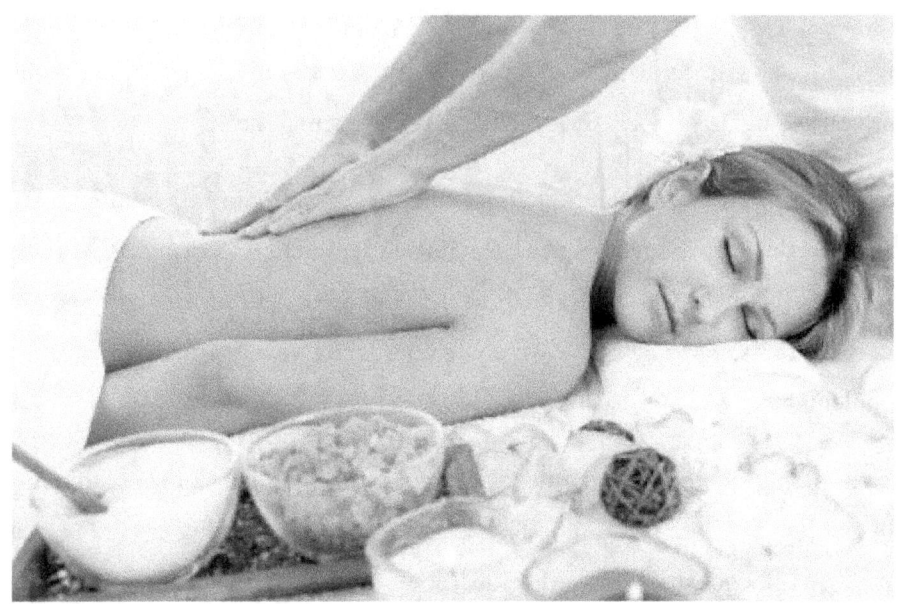

Massage is a noninvasive healing therapeutic technique, which helps strengthen tissue, and relax you.

If you want to know more about massage, here is a link to one of our publications.

Knowing More about Self Massage - http://tinyurl.com/ze8k33r

The best massage, done traditionally is of course the one which you do on your own body, by your own hands. That is because all your pressure points are gaining complete benefit by pressing on other pressure points on your body. This is going to increase the state of good health and well-being in your body, especially when you find it relaxing through the healing power of touch.

Neck Massage

Here are the usual massage methods which I use especially when I am feeling tense, and want to get rid of the knots at the back of my neck. For a rough massage, I just roll up a towel. If you want a really soft and gentle massage, twist three soft scarves together and make a thick braided shape. Put the scarves behind your neck with one hand holding one end each. Then do the rubbing in the tense area, so that tension is released and you can relax.

This reminds me of a scene in the blockbuster movie, <u>Pride and Prejudice,</u> when the hero Martin Henderson – "Mister Darcy" finds himself taking part in an Indian wedding scene. According to him, what are the dance movements, just put an invisible towel behind your neck, and shift it from right to left, while shifting the rest of your body. The next dance technique, according to him is changing a lightbulb with one uplifted hand while petting the dog with the other!

Incidentally, this movie was released when my cousin was married in a totally traditional wedding ceremony, where the clan gathered together the night before the ceremony to eat, drink, and dance the whole night through.

And just for fun, being the eldest sister of the family, I was asked to dance – no member is exempt from dancing from grand parents and relatives to grandchildren, any who can toddle, yell, and shout and make a joyous noise, because this show of happiness is supposed to be the harbinger of good fortune and blessings on the couple – I had to do a bit of tinkle toe-ing.

So being a complete ham – I said, "gather all ye together and I am going to teach you how to dance in three simple steps.

Imaginary towel behind neck – I swung it into a airy roll and then wrapped it over my head, positioning it behind my neck, while my 88-year-old grandmother – her grand aunt – and all the rest of the elders sat there and enjoyed the fun – shift the body to left and shift body to right, while massaging the back of the neck with this towel, check out the hand movements."

It was a riot! When everybody had stopped giggling, they all joined in, even those who were too shy to dance, because here was one relative having plenty of fun without even being self-conscious. After the bulb changing and dog patting session was over, everybody decided that this was an excellent way in which one could learn how to dance.

So you are going to be using a real towel/scarves and let the fun begin. *Owey-Owey -yah.Ohey- Ohey- yo!*

So this is for the neck. Now we come to the upper back.

Upper Back Massage

You will need a tennis ball here, which you are going to place between the area between the shoulder blade and your spine, and the wall. Just press the back into the tennis ball, shifting your body in such a manner that the spine is not pressed into the ball. You can either do up/down movements or you can do left and right movements. After sometime, shift to the area between the spine and the right blade of your shoulder.

Shoulder pain

Normally, I use a little bit of warm oil, to get rid of shoulder pain. I just dip the last three fingers in the oil and if I am massaging my left shoulder. I will be using my left hand. Cover the shoulder muscles, especially the aching area and do a little bit of massaging/pressing/squeezing with your fingers. Rotate your head from side to side at the same time, thus loosening the painful muscles around your neck at the same time.

If you are rolling your fingers or knuckles over the tissue, make sure it is done in the direction of your neck base, from the outside inwards.

You are going to use your right hand on your right shoulder with the palm covering the upper trapezius.

If you are suffering from lower back pain, and there is no medical reason for it, you may ask a qualified physiotherapist about a self massage system which works for you. The only lower back self massage method which I use is just using a little bit of traditional Tiger balm – this is an alternative medicine originally made somewhere in Singapore, – and massaging the affected area in circular motions for a couple of minutes until the pain goes away.

There are plenty of handheld massagers also available easily in the market today, and most of them are battery operated.

HoMedics is a good company and mine is the contour point handheld full-body massager with heat – Thera P. Though I have never used it! For me, when I have to massage and get rid of the stress in my neck muscles and shoulder muscles, I use my fingers and palms. Let me tell you the funny reason I do not use this massager. The moment I switch it on, the massager begins to go whirrr like a crazy bumblebee, and makes contact with any part of my body, I jump out of my skin! I just do not like that particular pressure and noise on my pressure points. Ah well! On the other hand , the rest of the family loves it!

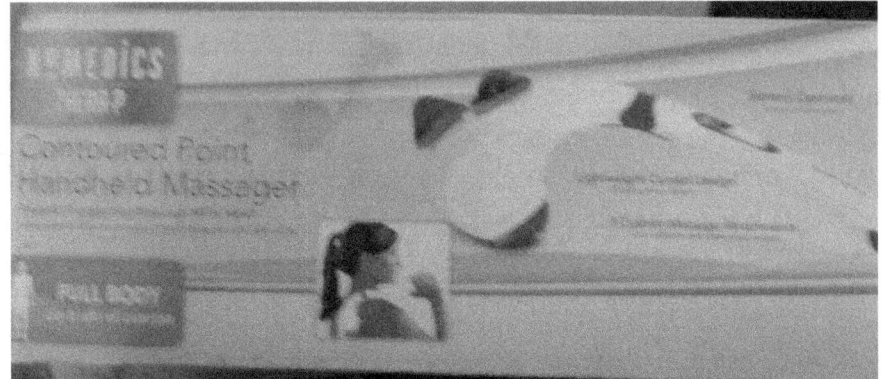

Conclusion

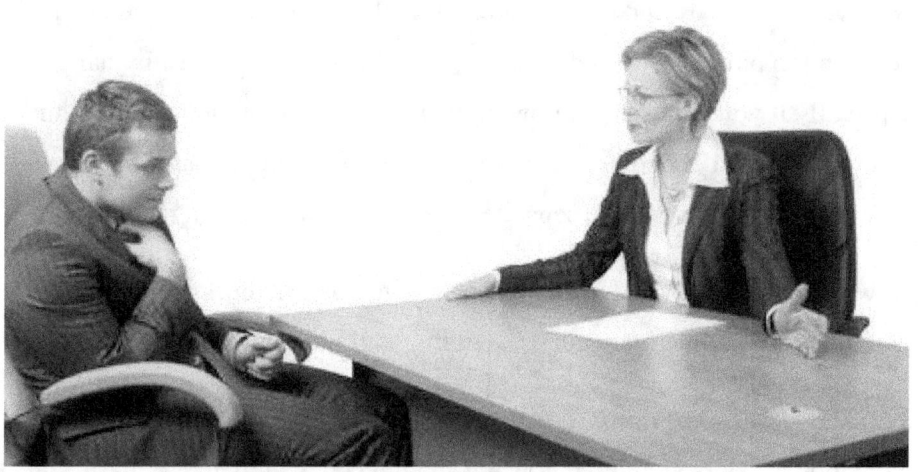

Look at the hunched shoulders and bad posture.

This book has given you plenty of information about how you can prevent backaches, especially through correct posture, massage, diet, and a change in your lifestyle.

Anyway, coming back to posture, if you find yourself suffering from rounded shoulders, like I did at college – I use to hunch in order to hide my six-foot height in a place where the average height of men was 5 foot six – seven and women was 5 foot four… The correction is not going to lie here in throwing your shoulders back and standing up straight – unless you want them straightened out with a military rattan cane – but here you are going to get your whole body back into line.

Stand in front of a mirror. Your feet should be about 6 inches apart and your toes should point straight ahead. The knees should be slightly relaxed and the arms should hang naturally, by your sides.

Now you are slowly and steadily going to pull your stomach in and up. You are going to pull your behind in and down. This is going to be a bit hard, especially if you are used to allowing your stomach to fall hither and thither and where it will. Stand as tall as you can, lifting the upper part of your body as though you want to separate it from the lower part, at the waistline.

Now, hold your head and neck high as though you are settling the back of your neck on an imaginary collar or tilting your chin and your nose at an imaginary foe.

Now look at yourself and see how the shoulders have fallen into place, and adjusted themselves naturally. If your shoulders are really rounded, stand with your head, arms, and the shoulders drooping forwards and limply. Now raise the upper part of the body, pulling in the stomach muscles. At the same time, you are going to draw your chest/bust upwards and raise the arms sideways. The shoulders are going to be high with your arms relaxed and the elbows slightly bent. Keep your palms up. Now you are going to drop your head backwards. Make sure that the shoulders are not hunched when you are doing this exercise. Go to the beginning and repeat again a number of times to straighten your rounded shoulders.

Incidentally, I talked about the model walk, walking from the hips, on an imaginary line. You can also try out this way to find out how you walk and whether your posture is proper. Put a really heavy book on the back of your head, and then try to cross the room. If the book stays on your head, congratulations, you are walking with natural balance and grace. If you find yourself with the book falling off, you will have to practice walking until you have learned how to keep it there.

My grandmother taught me to walk with three books balanced on my head for at least 10 minutes a day until I could balance them perfectly. Incidentally, at this time, we were living in a desert area where women walked 10 miles every day to a water source in order to get some water. And I must say, that I have never seen anyone more graceful and queenlier than those ladies, with their clay earthenware pots balanced perfectly on their heads, walking without spilling a drop or holding it in place.

In the same way, when you sit down make sure that you do not loll in an ungraceful posture, with the weight of the body on the small of your backs, sitting with your feet spread apart. Rather unattractive. And when you stand up, if you find yourself with your legs far apart as if you are bracing yourself on the deck of a ship with a hurricane coming on, or walk with your feet turned in slightly like a pigeon does, remember that these actions can either be a thing of beauty or quite the opposite.

Remember to choose a chair, which is straight back-ed. When you sit on it, sit up with the back straight and your feet crossed, 1 foot slightly behind the other and your knees leaning in one direction. You will be surprised at the feeling of natural poise, which a good posture can give you. Practice this until it becomes unconscious and habitual.

So remember that backaches are a thing which can be avoided, with just a little bit of effort.

Live Long and Prosper!

Author Bio

Dueep Jyot Singh is a Management and IT Professional who managed to gather Postgraduate qualifications in Management and English and Degrees in Science, French and Education while pursuing different enjoyable career options like being an hospital administrator, IT,SEO and HRD Database Manager/ trainer, movie , radio and TV scriptwriter, theatre artiste and public speaker, lecturer in French, Marketing and Advertising, ex-Editor of Hearts On Fire (now known as Solstice) Books Missouri USA, advice columnist and cartoonist, publisher and Aviation School trainer, ex-moderator on Medico.in, banker, student councilor ,travelogue writer … among other things!

One fine morning, she decided that she had enough of killing herself by Degrees and went back to her first love -- writing. It's more enjoyable! She already has 48 published academic and 14 fiction- in- different- genre books under her belt.

When she is not designing websites or making Graphic design illustrations for clients , she is browsing through old bookshops hunting for treasures, of which she has an enviable collection – including R.L. Stevenson, O.Henry, Dornford Yates, Maurice Walsh, De Maupassant, Victor Hugo, Sapper, C.N. Williamson, "Bartimeus" and the crown of her collection- Dickens "The Old Curiosity Shop," and "Martin Chuzzlewit" and so on… Just call her "Renaissance Woman" - collecting herbal remedies, acting like Universal Helping Hand/Agony Aunt, or escaping to her dear mountains for a bit of exploring, collecting herbs and plants, and trekking.

Check out some of the other JD-Biz Publishing books

Gardening Series on Amazon

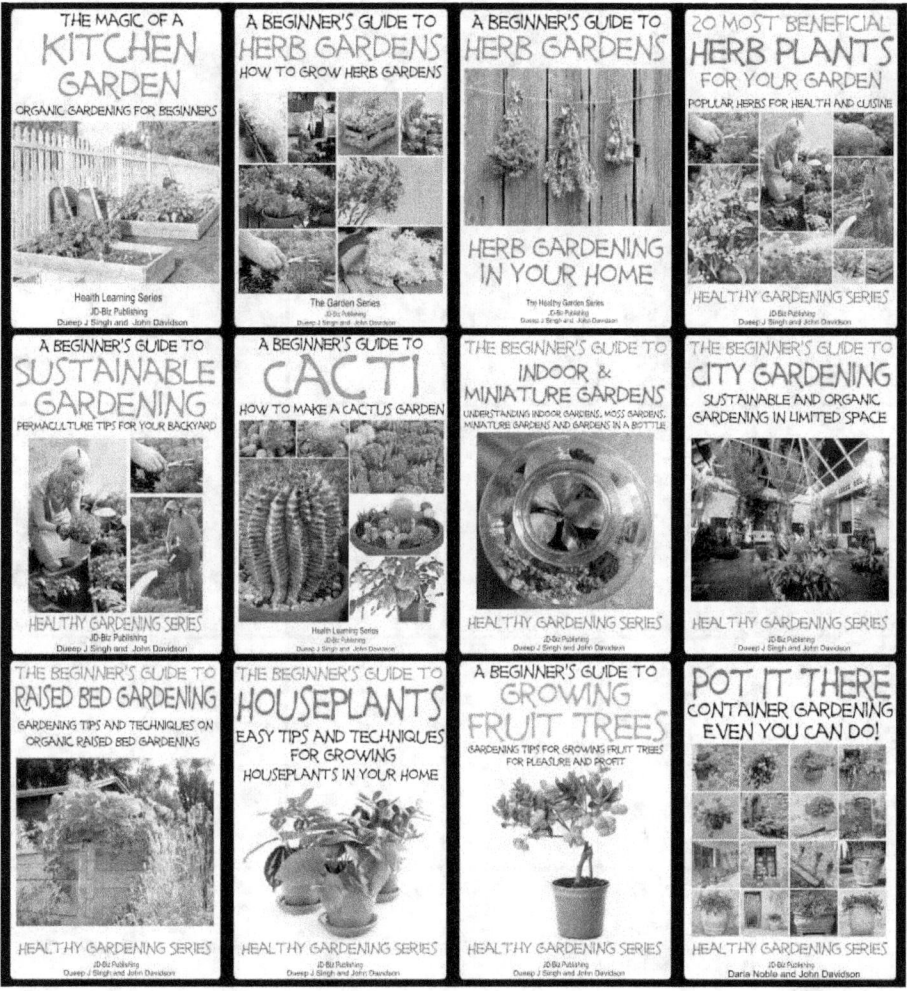

Download Free Books!

http://MendonCottageBooks.com

Health Learning Series

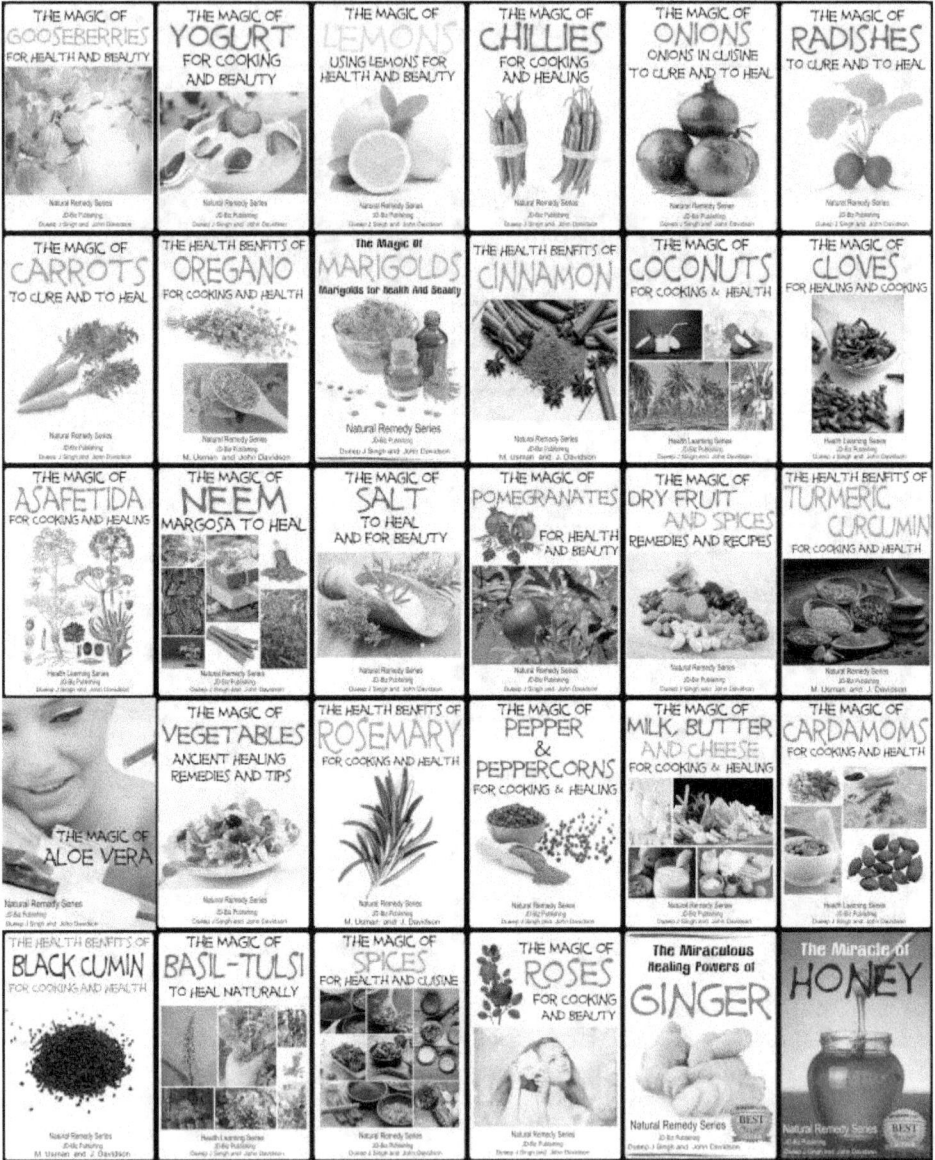

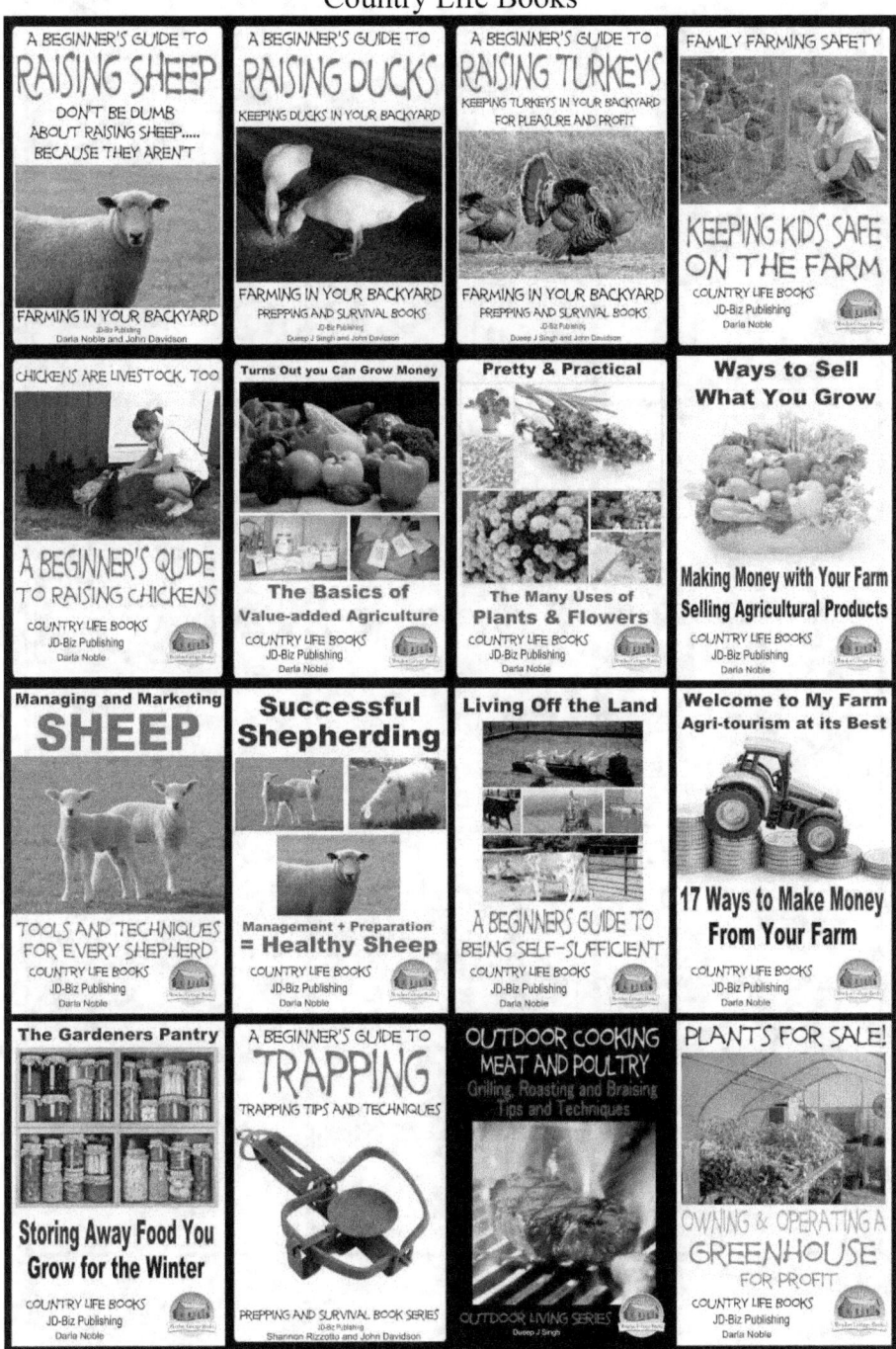

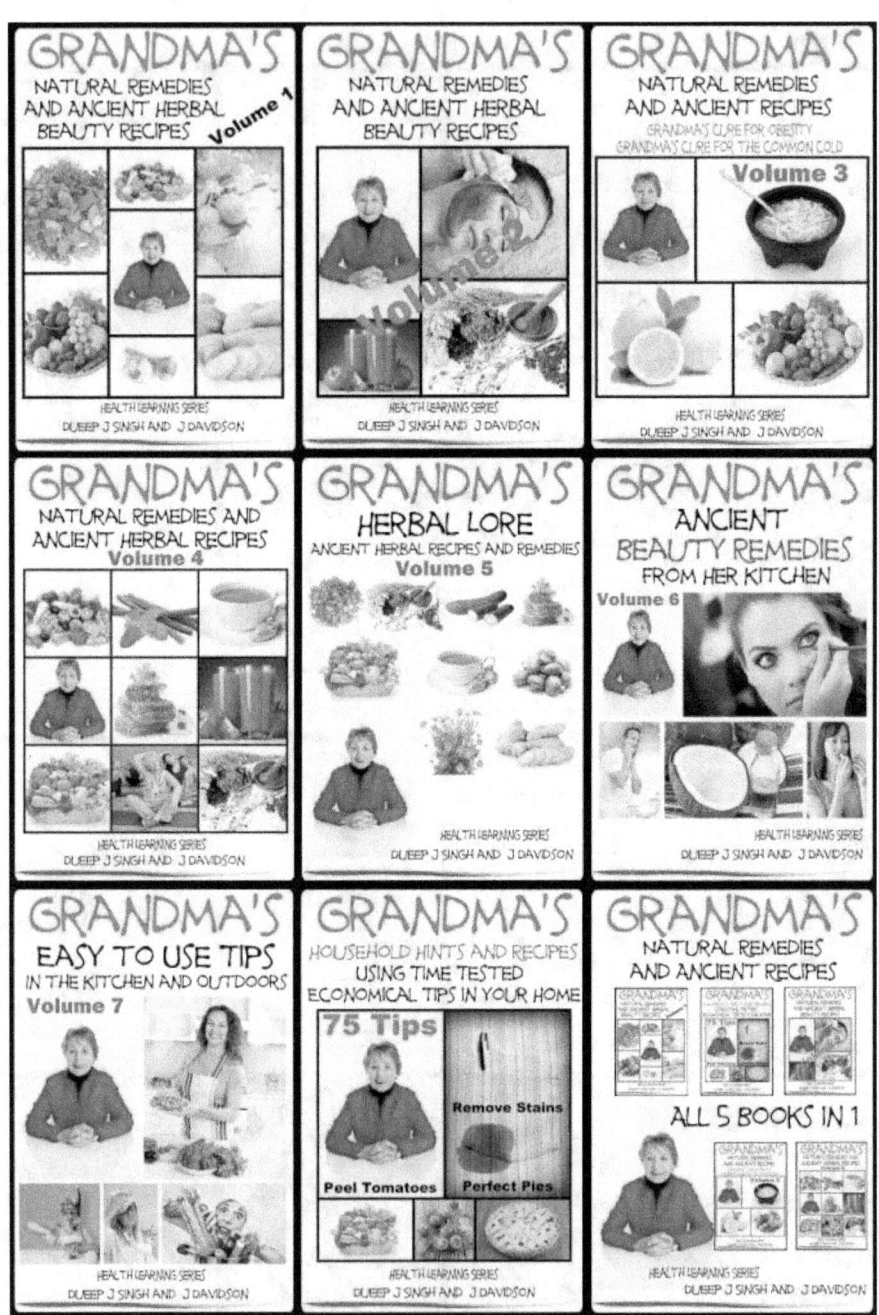

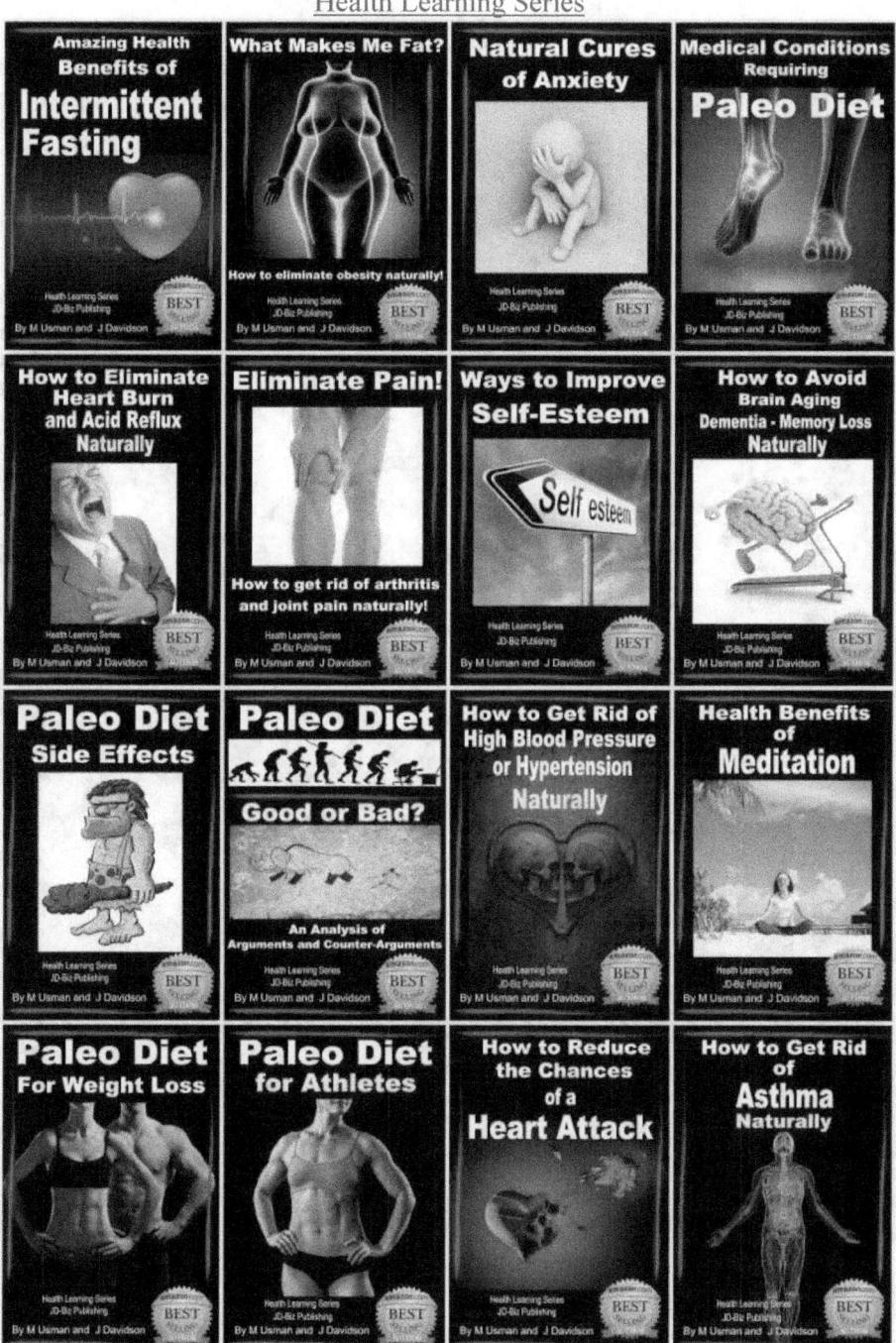

Amazing Animal Book Series

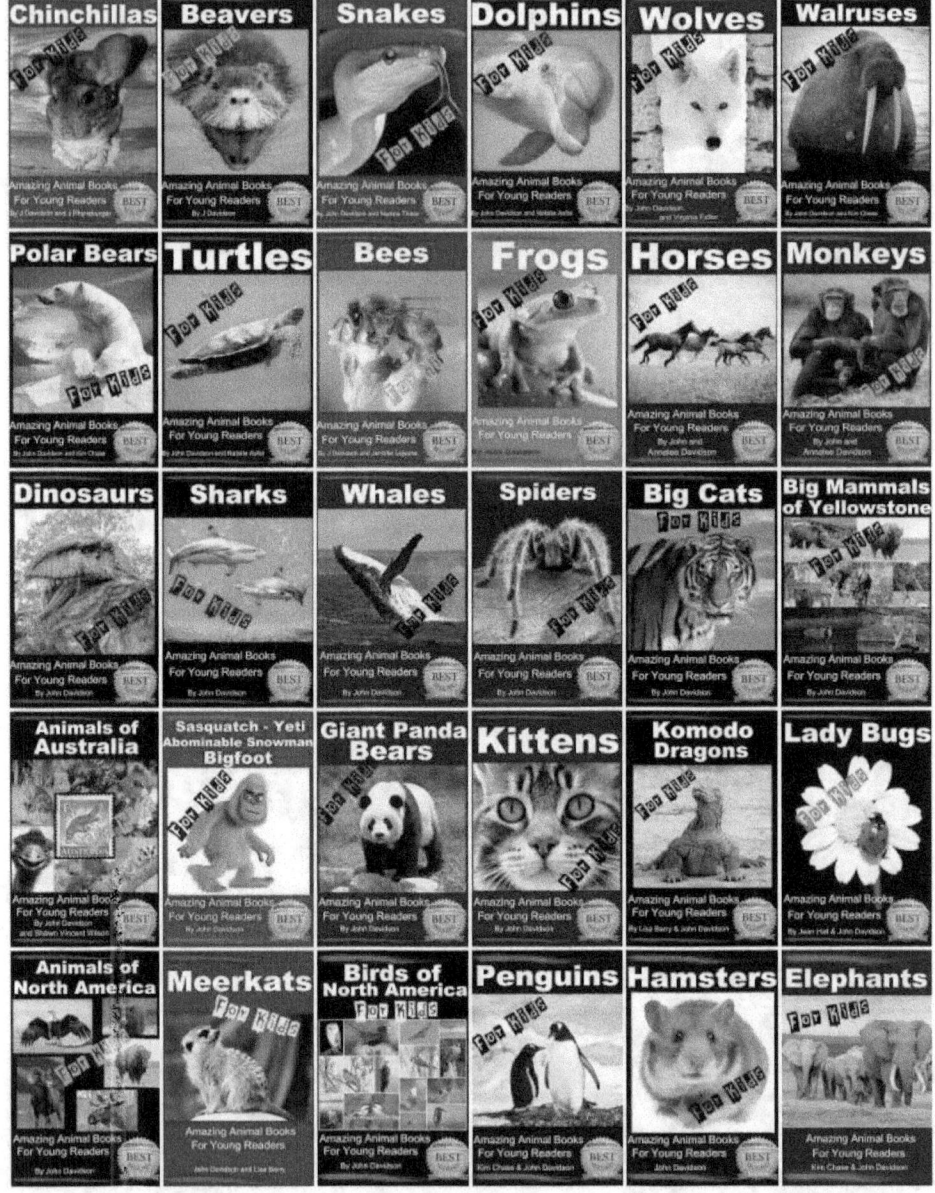

Learn To Draw Series

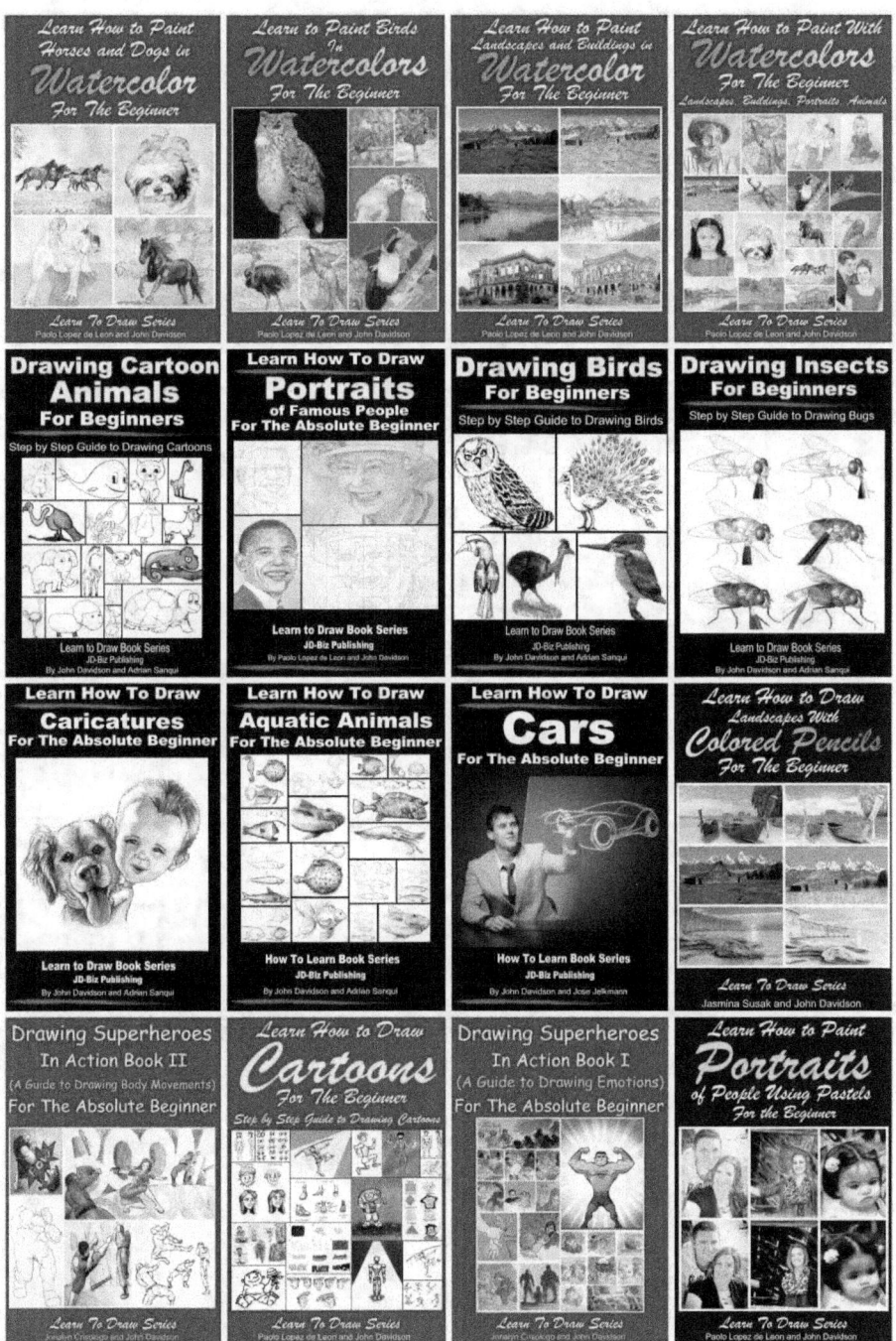

How to Build and Plan Books

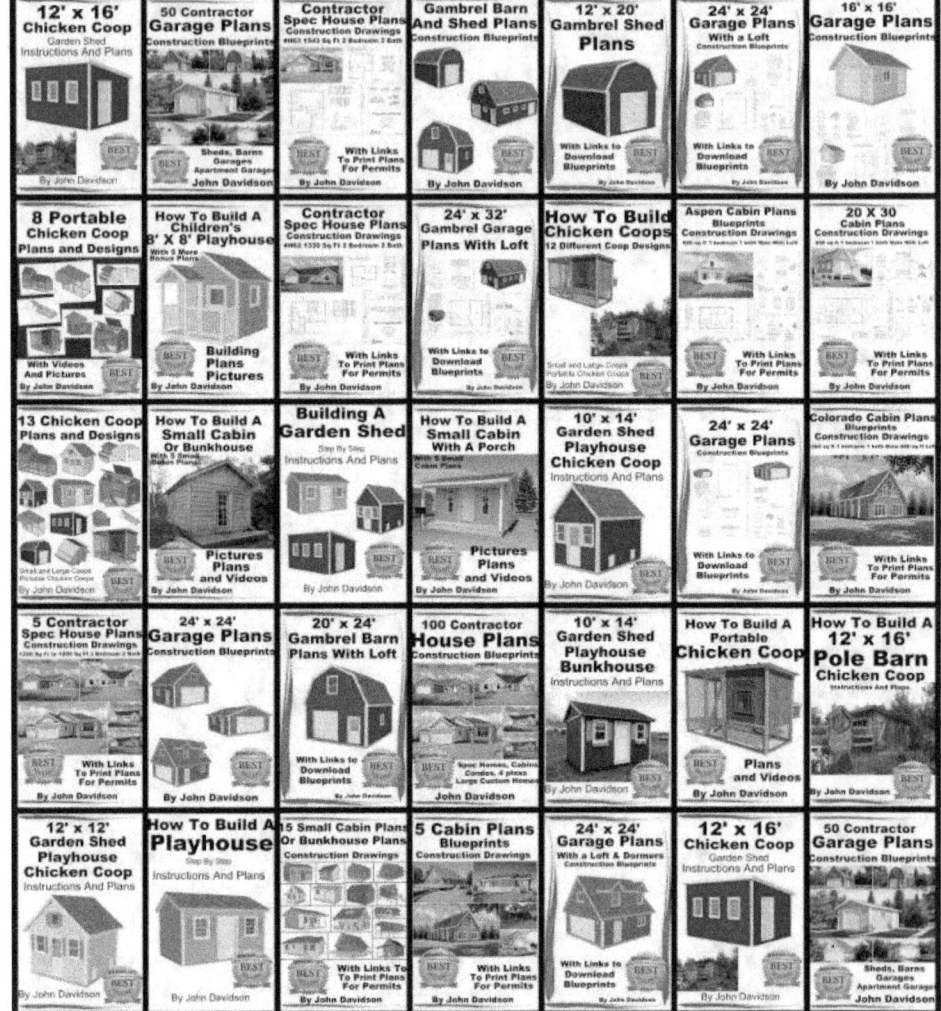

Entrepreneur Book Series

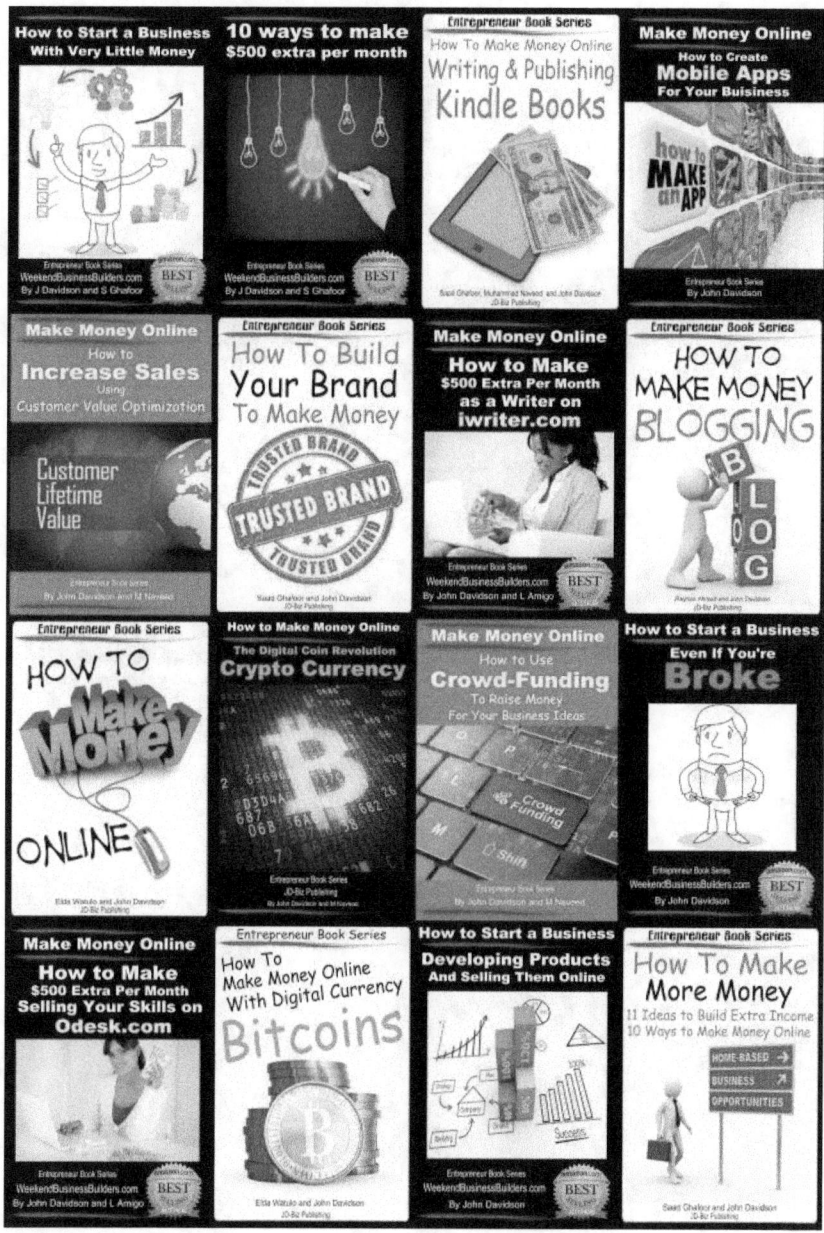

Our books are available at

1. Amazon.com

2. Barnes and Noble

3. Itunes

4. Kobo

5. Smashwords

6. Google Play Books

Download Free Books!

http://MendonCottageBooks.com

Publisher

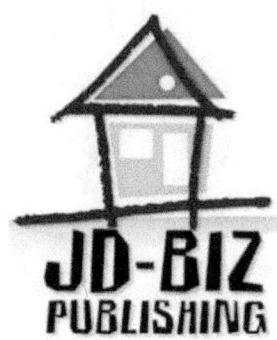

JD-Biz Corp

P O Box 374

Mendon, Utah 84325

http://www.jd-biz.com/

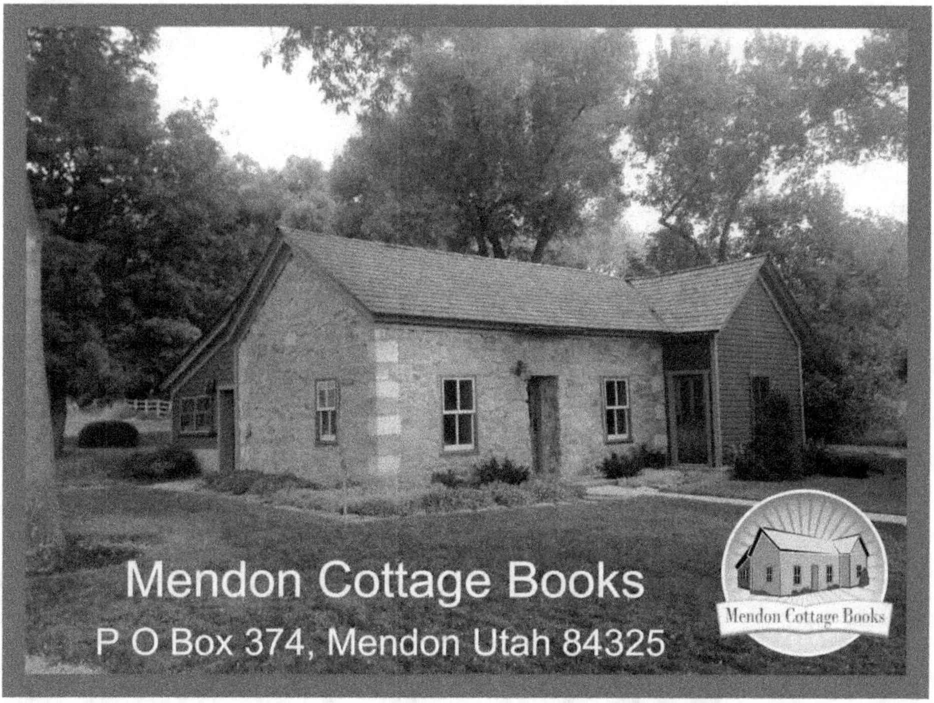

Mendon Cottage Books

P O Box 374, Mendon Utah 84325

Mendon Cottage Books